HEALTHCARE, ACTUALLY

A Brief Review of International Healthcare,
America's Challenges, and Steps Towards
Universal Healthcare

Jon Wees

First paperback edition May 2020

Book design by Autumn Gerfen

ISBN 978-1-7339904-0-0 (paperback)
ISBN 978-1-7339904-1-7 (ebook)

Published by Jon Wees
jhwees@gmail.com

INTRODUCTION

As someone who has worked in healthcare for a decade, when I've talked to my peers (millennials and Gen Y) over the past few years, hearing them speak about healthcare reform seems like it will be a miraculous transformation. Insurance coverage for every individual across all walks of life so no one goes bankrupt from bills. No treatment beyond the reach of patients to access or doctors to prescribe. With a stroke of a pen, legislation will improve the lives of millions instantly. What they describe *is* a fantasy. The healthcare industry is one-fifth (20%) of our national economy. The stone-cold truth is we can't transform this nation overnight. Expansive healthcare reform, when it comes, will be arduous, nuanced, time-consuming, and exhausting - exactly like the Affordable Care Act was (ACA).

And the United States, no matter how often We the People call for it, is not ready or willing to institute single-payer. Regardless of what political power is in charge, the reality of the nation - economically, industrially, socially - doesn't permit single-payer at this time. It's certainly an ideal, an aspiration to work towards, but it's not the only option. It's also, despite common opinion, not what most nations use as their healthcare infrastructure.

Before we continue, let's introduce some definitions to this conversation:

- **Single-payer healthcare:** a national health insurance program run and financed by the central/federal government *only*, rather than by regional or private insurers, to cover all healthcare costs
- **Universal healthcare:** a national health insurance program designed by the government to regulate and/or provide health care and financial protection to all citizens

Single-payer is universal healthcare; but not all universal healthcare is single-payer. This is a subtle but important distinction, and the reason why I decided to write this book.

One day we may have a single-payer system. I am not naive enough to believe it'll happen in my lifetime. There are exceptional and, *nuanced* reasons why this is true, but that doesn't mean we as a nation cannot take the first steps towards single-payer for the future. In a way we already have, with the ACA providing a solid foundation. To go beyond that framework, however, we first have to know what options are out there, what hurdles stand in our way, and what we can do *now* to achieve our goal for *then*.

To that end, this book is divided into three sections. The first is a brief examination of the systems of other nations with universal healthcare. The second is dedicated to the healthcare in the United States and why a single-payer healthcare system is a challenge to implement. The third is a series of proposals and suggestions ranging from the simple to the extreme that could lead the way to our own form of universal healthcare.

This is a short simple review of a highly complex and nuanced topic. By addressing these details even briefly I can hopefully provide some clarification of the challenges facing us nationally in healthcare reform. The goal here is to foster discussion and debate of the ideas on universal healthcare, and that there are many paths to it.

INTERNATIONAL SYSTEMS

When it comes to single-payer, everyone from politicians to vocal supporters to quiet commentators point to our international allies as examples of how it could be; of how much *better* their healthcare system is; how their citizens are happier, healthier, and more content when it comes to healthcare. They are, for the most part, correct. In fact, there are three near-universal social truths when it comes to successful universal healthcare programs across the world.

1) The people of the nation have come to a consensus that not only is healthcare a right, but that they have a responsibility to help make healthcare accessible for everyone

2) As a right granted to everyone, healthcare must be affordable so that no one goes bankrupt seeking treatment

3) To make healthcare affordable, it must be cost effective, so direct and indirect government regulation is required (i.e., the insurance market, negotiating prices with pharmaceutical companies, owning and operating medical facilities in the nation, etc.)

This last aspect, which we'll call **fettered capitalism** - constraining the hand of the free market - is a crucial component that stands out when compared to the American system. In the United States the free market is, to many, beyond reproach. It's why a CEO can purchase a small manufacturing company and increase the cost of a lifesaving drug to 500 times its current price. It's why insurance companies can set roadblocks to getting vital treatments and provide minimal coverage. It's why doctors can turn away desperate patients simply because they're on Medicaid. Examples are endless.

The Affordable Care Act (ACA) attempted to address some of these issues. A prime example is the regulation of minimum healthcare services covered by insurance companies. The expansion of Medicaid programs and willingness to work on unique models with states for maximum coverage is another. Before the ACA, the Child Health Insurance Plan, proposed and passed by President Clinton in the 1990s crossed the line of socialism by ensuring underprivileged children wouldn't be without healthcare; regardless of the free-market's situation. Medicare itself is a form of *fettered capitalism*, where the government regulates treatment and procedure prices across its network.

Unfortunately, all of these programs are susceptible to the whims of politics, courts, and the influence of big business. As long as we, as a nation, continue to ***not*** form a national consensus on how to handle healthcare, we'll be unable to pass any form of single-payer or universal healthcare plan without risk of it falling apart during the transition of power from one president or Congress to another.

This is not true with many healthcare programs around the world. They have accepted fettered capitalism as a necessary instrument to ensure no one is denied coverage and no one suffers financially simply for trying to stay alive. However there are some fundamental misconceptions Americans have regarding these healthcare programs. Before we can address what may work for healthcare reform in our nation, we must understand some truths about programs elsewhere.

In the following pages we'll review nine international healthcare systems, along with brief mentions of some additional ones. Included with the details of each nation's systems will be their population, gross domestic product (GDP), and land area; along with the ratio between that data and the United States. This information is included primarily to point out a direct one-to-one comparison for implementing healthcare systems in the US isn't necessarily appropriate. Whenever a program grows or expands exponentially the more complicated and complex that program becomes. In other words, what works in a nation that is exponentially smaller (demographically, financially, geographically) may not easily extrapolate to a successful model when applied to the United States.

This is perhaps best exemplified by the smaller nations sometimes quoted as excellent models for the United States to follow: **Denmark, Israel, New Zealand, Norway, Sweden, and Switzerland.** These nations may at first seem to be completely unrelated to each other but there are three details that matter for this review: each of these nations has less than 10 million in population; is no larger than 200,000 square miles; and none have a gross domestic product (GDP) above $700 billion. To put that into perspective, none of these nations are larger than the state of Montana, all have less than New Jersey's population, and all make no more than Ohio's GDP.

What they do have is their own version of universal healthcare. While these systems are successful and well-designed, they are also systems successful on a small-scale. These systems work now because they are in a contained area with a low, homogenized (except Israel) population generating a high enough GDP able to address and cover the concerns of healthcare. Nigeria, which has both a comparable area and GDP but exponentially higher population (at almost 200 million), has a universal healthcare system set up. It is not nearly as successful because population is dramatically increased, resulting in approximately 50% of the inhabitants - the urban inhabitants - having access to the nation's universal healthcare system and rural areas lacking accessibility and infrastructure.

Therefore these smaller nations are not excellent examples of how to implement national healthcare. If anything, they prove that single states - Texas, California, New York - have models to emulate. The downside is that the states most likely to implement such models would be those with Democratically controlled legislatures, resulting in an even greater inequality of healthcare coverage from state to state. This acute political division of healthcare at the state level could even be a hindrance in creating a national healthcare system.

Nonetheless, there are some details about these international plans worth looking at when trying to improve our own healthcare system.

- **Denmark:** Citizens are automatically enrolled in their universal healthcare system, but there is a private fund from doctors, the Red Cross, and nonprofits to help pay for the healthcare of visitors and undocumented immigrants. In addition, for the chronically ill, their pharmaceutical co-payments are reduced because their costs are higher. In other words, a patient with Multiple Sclerosis or cancer gets reimbursed for the cost of their high-priced, on-going treatments necessary to live, in an effort to alleviate the cost burden.

- **Israel:** If employers have non-citizens in their nation, it is the employer's responsibility to enroll its employees into private healthcare with equivalent coverage to the National Health Insurance guidelines for Israel, and to meet those guidelines this must be at no or minimal cost to the patient
- **New Zealand:** Copayments for prescribed drugs are required per family per year for the first 20 prescriptions, and then no further copayments for any drugs until the next year.
- **Norway:** Home-based and institutional care coverage is based on means testing – that is, based on a patient or family's annual income - and cost up to 85% of patient's personal income
- **Sweden:** Coverage copayments are set by local regions, and can include a subsidy where the government covers a certain amount financially, after which cost falls to the patient. This individual out-of-pocket cost is capped based on age and type of service (medical, dental, prescription).
- **Switzerland:** Insurance is mandatory and must be purchased by the patient (and for their dependents), often separate from their employer, from a nonprofit insurance company. This includes a minimum annual deductible, coinsurance, copayments, and an out-of-pocket cap on cost-sharing. Private insurance as a supplement is available, through price-regulated for-profit entities. Dentistry and long-term care are not part of the mandatory covered systems.

Another small nation's healthcare system worth mentioning is **Singapore**, which has a very different type of universal healthcare. While it has the government regulation (*fettered capitalism*) of public and private insurance of the other smaller nations above, it tries to match that regulation with public responsibility. Each citizen has a mandatory health savings account (HSA) to help offset medical expenses by deducting wages into this dedicated account. They also have a secondary healthcare fund to help with catastrophic medical treatment, such as long-term illness (i.e., cancer) that the HSA might not be able to cover. There is a government fund to cover the costs of those unable to afford treatment through the first two funds. Finally, there is private insurance to augment the first two personal funds as well.

It's worth mentioning these mandated funds because this is often the Conservative argument for health saving funds (HSA) in the United States - personal and financial responsibility for one's health. These same Americans advocate for HSA while tending to neglect the role of the federal government needed to offset the potential high costs of medical care by having strict cost regulation and subsidizing of medical care, in Singapore's case this is approximately 80%. Should America embrace national HSAs, it should be noted that half of the program alone is not enough, and cost regulation is needed for success in both the public and private sector.

Having identified what quoted nations are *not* excellent models, let's continue with the nations supporters of single-payer healthcare most commonly reference: **Canada, Australia, and the United Kingdom.** Though they loom large on the international political stage and in the arguments of single-payer advocates, the statistics and details will show there are dramatic differences in population, GDP, and/or geography that mean those systems might not work for the US. They are still, however, systems worth examining as models to build off from.

Canada

Let's begin with the first misconception: this is not a true single-payer system. Each Province -

Population	37.1 million (2018)	11.3% of US
GDP	$1.71 trillion (2018)	8.3% of US
Land Area	3.855 million sq mi	100.1% of US

British Columbia, Quebec, etc. -administers, regulates, funds, and sets reimbursement for their own versions of universal healthcare. These Provinces must follow a federal mandate called the Canadian Healthcare Act to get a percentage of federal funds to complement their own funding systems. The federal government also handles safety and efficacy, to ensure the quality of any pharmaceuticals, medical devices, and treatment itself is equal across the Provinces. There is no program to enroll in; citizens of Canada are simply covered by their Provincial healthcare.

The other common myth is that this program covers everything, and that taxes are the only cost-sharing a patient faces. This is also incorrect. Dental care, vision care, non-hospital prescriptions, rehabilitation, and home care are *not* included in the Canadian Healthcare Act. There are also additional patient liabilities from Province to Province. For instance, in Ontario a ride in an ambulance is *not* covered by the universal healthcare plan. These are all subject to patient out-of-pocket expenditures in addition to the taxes paid.

Instead, Canada turns to for-profit insurance companies who cover these gaps. Much like the United States, many companies offer this private insurance as an employee perk deducted from their paycheck. In addition to the above, these plans can include a private room during a hospital stay, ambulance rides, and in some cases more non-standard services such as acupuncture. So, while many would espouse Canada is the perfect single-payer, it does include a massive private insurance industry that two-thirds of the citizens are enrolled in.

The difference is that Canada believes in *fettered capitalism,* and these for-profit companies work within the Canadian price-limitation regulations. Even without private insurance, though, costs are lower than in America thanks to Canada's federal government. There is a federal review board that sets prices for drugs - brand and generic - and negotiates directly with the pharmaceutical companies. Either drug companies accept the negotiated contracted price, or they don't sell any drugs in the Province. Between some market share or none at all, many companies accept the limitation. This body also sets fee schedules - reimbursement - for doctors and their services, along with limits on the number of doctors and nurses permitted on facility budgets.

Australia

Much like Canada, the funding and administration of this universal healthcare system is done

Population	24.9 million (2018)	7.6% of US
GDP	$1.43 trillion (2018)	7% of US
Land Area	2.97 million sq mi	78% of US

regionally, with some matching funds from their federal government. And like Canada, dental, vision, ambulance, and some prescriptions are not covered under their universal healthcare program. There are, however, some vast differences.

There are two healthcare programs: the well-known Medicare for medical coverage, and the lesser-known Pharmaceutical Benefit program, covering pharmaceuticals. Medicare in Australia, though sharing a name with a United States program, is drastically different from both its American counterpart, and from Canada's universal coverage program. Where Canada does not allow doctors to charge more than the schedule fee set in their Provincial guidelines, Australia allows doctors to request reimbursement above their fees if the Medicare or Pharmaceutical programs don't reimburse at 100%. As an example, General Practitioners (GP) are covered at 100% of reimbursement, but specialists at only 85%, and either can request more than that reimbursement amount be paid (although 80% of GPs don't make that request).

Another difference is that while Canada does not actively promote or encourage its citizens to get private health insurance, Australia does. In fact, it has a thriving for-profit (and nonprofit) insurance industry complementing its federal programs. These insurance programs allow for faster access to services, greater choice of doctors, dentistry, vision, chiropractic, and other services. The government encourages people to enroll in these private programs through a tax rebate and, if an individual has a higher income, a tax penalty for *not* enrolling.

Unlike the United States, however, these private insurance companies have their maximum reimbursement rates set to the Medicare and Pharmaceutical program rate, i.e., the insurance covers 85% of the Medicare reimbursement and no more. It is up to the patient to pay this difference; but insurances and medical facilities are encouraged not to inflate these costs as there is also a maximum annual out-of-pocket cost after which patients are covered 100%, a detail the ACA tried to mimic. Similarly, medications and some medical services have a maximum annual out-of-pocket based on patient income, after which their costs are set - no higher or lower - for the rest of the year, also based on their income.

Australia also has a universal electronic patient record system. Canada has Provincial electronic records, but they are not required to be transmittable from one Province to another. Australia, on the other hand, has not only a national database, but it is designed to be accessible by doctors, insurers, and patients themselves, including the self-input of end-of-care directives if so desired.

United Kingdom

This is perhaps the closest to an actual single-payer healthcare system that exists on this

Population	66.4 million (2018)	20.3% of US
GDP	$2.83 trillion (2018)	13.8% of US
Land Area	93,628 sq mi	2.5% of US

most-quoted list. Personal and corporate taxes contribute to this single healthcare system, the National Healthcare System (NHS), that oversees not only medical coverage, but dental, vision, ambulance, and almost every other medical and pharmaceutical service available. This coverage is free, for the most part, and formerly included not only British citizens, but any European Union card carrying member prior to the country's departure from the E.U.

The biggest myth is that this is all "free" to the patient. There is, however, actual cost-sharing for the patients, save children and the elderly. Some prescription drugs, dentistry services, and long-term care are subject to co-payments. Once again *fettered capitalism* comes into play, as copayments are set on the national level and doctors are not allowed to charge more than these amounts. Long-term and residential care, it should be noted, also has cost-sharing requirements based on income, and can be more than the government limit due to the quality and private institutions available for patients.

Finally, in addition to the private institutions for long-term care, there is private insurance available to purchase. These exclude any maternity, mental health, emergency and general care. Instead these private insurances are for expedited and more convenient access to care, primarily for elective hospital procedures. This market, however, is exceptionally small at approximately 10% of the population (as of 2016), and while regulated, is obviously a minority consideration to the majority of the nation's population.

Costs are contained by a national budget, which sets salaries for doctors, negotiates costs for pharmaceuticals, and sets fees for hospitals. This is the closest thing to our definition of a single-payer system, and the one *least* likely to occur in the United States. American doctors already do not like the Medicare/Medicaid federal and state-mandated reimbursement rates. Many would refuse to become government employees. While the prices and ease of access is alluring for the American public, the logistics, administration and cognitive mental shift that would be required both within the healthcare profession and by the US population would be enormous. And, as proven by the NHS and its financial difficulties, this model is subject to the whims of political pressure and changes, to the detriment of the system and the people.

Aspects of both Canada and Australia's universal healthcare programs seem like they'd be an easy accommodation for the United States to adopt. Unfortunately, the mindset of politicians and some citizens say otherwise. As of 2017, there are still 19 state houses that refuse to expand their Medicaid coverage - despite citizens of those states demanding expanded coverage. When the ACA attempted to enforce and regulate minimum coverage requirements for insurances a number of states, companies, and religious institutions sued, objecting to the contraception provisions. Insurance companies are now fighting against the regulation that women cannot be charged more than men for healthcare insurance. ***Unless and until the federal government and Supreme Court are willing to declare healthcare a right and not a privilege, on par with the First Amendment, any form of universal healthcare is unlikely to come about.***

There are not, however, only three nations to look at for inspiration to build universal healthcare. I want to now address some of the least talked about national healthcare systems, but some of the ones that are perhaps most important in terms of determining the next evolution for healthcare in the United States: **France, Germany, Italy, Japan, and Spain**. These nations not only use *fettered capitalism*, they have one or all of the three variables - population, size, and GDP - that are not exponentially smaller, but only by an order of magnitude - i.e., half the population, one quarter of the GDP, etc. These are healthcare programs that may not directly translate to the US, but they may be more accessible in establishing a national US system.

France

Not counting the United States, France has the highest cost of healthcare per capita

Population	65 million (2018)	19.9% of US
GDP	$2.78 trillion (2018)	13.6% of US
Land Area	248,537 sq mi	6.5% of US

of all developed nations with universal healthcare. Having a similar single-payer model to the United Kingdom, all medical services, drugs, and reimbursement rates are set at the national level, including transportation and partial coverage for long-term services. Unlike the United Kingdom, however, coverage is minimal for dental and vision services; and patients help cover the costs both of the programs and physician reimbursement through co-insurances and copayments rather than taxes. These costs are set by France's physician's union that negotiates their reimbursement with the government (it should be noted that US law prohibits physicians from forming unions). In addition, especially for vision and dental, nonprofit insurance companies offer complimentary coverage that patients and companies can purchase.

Compared to the other nations reviewed, the French government has a more active financial role with both physicians and patients. The government incentivizes doctors to care for chronic patients with extra reimbursement, and to ensure national healthcare coverage guarantees a monthly income to those physicians who set up practice in regions with low physician accessibility. On the patient side, the government provides the elderly with means-tested monetary allowances to help with long-term care costs, and informal caregivers of these patients - i.e., adults caring for elderly parents - can apply for a tax break.

Germany

Similarly to Switzerland, insurance is mandatory for citizens to purchase

Population	83.1 million (2018)	25.4% of US
GDP	$4.01 trillion (2018)	19.6% of US
Land Area	137,983 sq mi	3.6% of US

and competing nonprofit insurance companies provide the majority of coverage. That's where the similarities end. Unlike the others, the German government takes little to no direct steps towards funding their universal healthcare system, focusing instead on regulation and keeping costs affordable (not excessive) for patients. Even when it comes to covering children and individuals of low-income, the government will only subsidize some of the nonprofit insurances - sickness funds - to step into the role of covering those individuals.

Instead of the government, the primary funding for these nonprofits comes from a percentage of patient's gross wages up to a regulated ceiling meaning both employers and employees contribute approximately 15% of their wages to fund these nonprofits. This funding is pooled, and then redistributed to the nonprofits based on a complicated algorithm that includes age, sex, demographic, geography, and additional variables, all supervised by the government.

Private insurance outside the sickness funds is available, and like many other nations, is also highly regulated to ensure costs are not excessive. As a result, less than half are for-profit. Some of the sickness funds can negotiate directly with pharmaceutical companies and providers to maintain the competition between nonprofit costs, but still under monitoring and regulation by the government to ensure no excessive costs to the patients. There is also a wage requirement: those who make less than a certain amount per year are not allowed to purchase private insurance and must remain in the public (nonprofit) system. Unlike most of the other nations reviewed, long-term care is required as part of Germany's healthcare coverage. Employer contributions to help fund these nonprofit insurance programs is mandatory.

It's important to note Germany has also moved away from fee-based reimbursement, and instead focuses on quality and efficacy; meaning "low-value" services are reimbursed less - no $200 fee for "Kleenex disposal" allowed. If this sounds familiar, the ACA implemented a similar protocol, though it's still being developed and balanced with the fee-based reimbursement system still in place.

Italy

This nation is very alike to Canada's system, with the federal government collecting taxes,

Population	60.6 million (2018)	18.5% of US
GDP	$2.07 trillion (2018)	10.1% of US
Land Area	116,347 sq mi	3.1% of US

distributing the funds to regions, and those regions working on the administration. Unlike Canada, procuring additional funding through regional taxes is optional, not required. There is also cost-sharing, as copayments are a standard part of procedures and pharmaceuticals. These copayments often have a maximum cap on cost per procedure, but not on the number of procedures so an office visit and x-ray will be billed separately and have two copays toward the national maximum.

This cost-sharing system is an important detail of their system, as there is no out-of-pocket cap to help protect patient expenses. Instead, when patients meet a national out-of-pocket annual limit, they are offered a tax credit to help offset those expenses. This is similar to the United States tax credit, though in the US it is based on a percentage of a person's income rather than Italy's flat national out-of-pocket amount.

Most of Italy's population is covered by the national insurance described above, and there is also some private insurance, typically for corporations and some non-corporate individuals. Some prescription drugs and dental services are not covered by the government plan with the typical exceptions (children, elderly, low-income), where the private insurance can step in. However, despite the direct negotiation and set reimbursement prices, Italy's healthcare system has a high debt, which has directly led to increases in copays across services. It should also be noted that drugs not directly negotiated with Italy but still available for use have costs set by the market, not government regulation, and contribute to patient out-of-pocket costs.

Japan

Japan is one of the least talked about universal healthcare systems in the world, but is one of the

Population	127.2 million (2018)	38.9% of US
GDP	$4.97 trillion (2018)	24.2% of US
Land Area	145,932 sq mi	3.8% of US

most important when examining how to expand healthcare in the United States. Unlike the three previously quoted (UK, Canada, Australia) Japan is more closely aligned with the US in terms of population (1/3rd of US) and GDP (1/4th of US). The greatest difficulty is in size, where the nation is comparable to the state of Montana. It's almost an amalgamation of many systems reviewed already, something that will also probably happen when universal healthcare takes form in the US.

To start with, Japan's Statutory Health Insurance System (SHIS) not only regulates medical and pharmaceutical costs, it sets a national fee schedule and provides subsidies to regional governments, insurance companies, and directly to doctors. Enrollment in one of the 3000-plus insurance plans is mandatory; but this provision is not strictly enforced as each prefecture has a "default" insurance choice that automatically covers its citizens. These are all public insurance plans, paid for per-household based on a percentage of annual income. Cost-sharing is a staple of this system, with an average coinsurance (patient cost) of 30% across most services.

Fettered capitalism steps in again as the Japanese government strictly regulates prices to ensure no excessive cost, and re-evaluates these prices every other year. Patients who spend above a certain out-of-pocket cost based on their annual income can include medical expenses as a tax deduction, much like in the United States. Monthly out-of-pocket limits are also set, which when met, reduce coinsurance to 1%, along with several other details in terms of catastrophic coverage to help keep patient costs down. An additional cost-saving measure is a law stating all hospitals must be nonprofit and all clinics must be owned by physicians. Patients over 40 also contribute towards a long-term care insurance in addition to their health insurance costs.

As you can see, there are aspects of many nations' healthcare systems within the Japanese system: Canada and France in how its funding is handled, competing insurance companies and mandatory long-term care contributions like Germany, cost-sharing with limits like Australia. Even the tax deduction similar to the United States. Japan has built a highly complex but effective system that, most importantly, they continue to improve upon for increased accessibility and public awareness of health initiatives.

Spain

Spain is the last system we'll be looking at closely, and has one unusual property compared

Population	46.7 million (2018)	14.3% of US
GDP	$1.43 trillion (2018)	7% of US
Land Area	195,364 sq mi	5.1% of US

to other national healthcare systems on this list: they have a divided healthcare system. A single-payer Spanish National Healthcare System (SNHS) covers the nation, along with regional healthcare run by autonomous communities. The Council of Spanish National Health ensures parity between these multiple systems. In the United States this would be comparable to California, New York, Washington, Texas, and Hawaii having state healthcare systems while all other states had Medicare for All.

In this unique model for healthcare, the SNHS sets forth its guidelines for minimal coverage, reimbursement rates, and financing guidelines. The autonomous communities then put out their own guidelines building off the SNHS guidelines but incorporating their own regional policies, such as extra taxes, fewer copays, or additional fee structures. That said, Spain's federal government has created a set of laws and rights of patients for healthcare access that both the nation and communities must follow. Payroll taxes have been phased out for funding, while indirect taxes (i.e., alcohol, tobacco, etc.) increased with a percentage dedicated to pay for healthcare.

Private insurance is available, much like it is in the United States, but it is more on par with the regulated pricing found in Europe and often is just a way to expand and expedite access to certain doctors or elective procedures. As a result, private insurance only covers approximately 19% of the population as of 2019. Copays are a part of the SNHS system, but is lower because of the national regulation on pricing. These prices can vary between SNHS and the autonomous communities, and as a result, has resulted in some prescription reimbursements taking years to fulfill due to the inter-committee bureaucracies.

While the SNHS is most similar to the UK's NHS system, the autonomous communities are more like the provinces of Canada, leaning more towards universal healthcare than single-payer. This could be a model to consider if some states in the US develop their own healthcare systems, which is why it's worth noting on this list. Whether that could lead to universal healthcare across the US, or set up funding fights as occasionally happen in Spain, is uncertain.

Though all of the above nations have less population than the US, there are two nations that have nearly four times the population of the US, one of which almost has the same land area; but neither are close to its GDP. I'm talking about **China and India,** and the challenges facing their healthcare systems.

Both nations have attempted to implement their own universal healthcare systems. While it seems such massive nations should be prime examples to follow, they both have serious issues to serve as warnings. The core issue is population density and accessibility of healthcare. Like the Nigeria example earlier, there isn't the infrastructure or enough doctors in either nation to provide sustainable healthcare.

China is taking steps towards reducing the disparity between urban and rural accessibility and private insurance

Nation	China	
Population	1.343 billion (2018)	410.6% of US
GDP	$13.6 trillion (2018)	60.3% of US
Land Area	3.71 million sq mi	97.7% of US

coverage, with most public plans covering a majority of medical and prescription costs. There is no uniformity across public plans, much less public and private.

India, on the other hand, leaves coverage and "right to life" healthcare to the individual states,

Nation	India	
Population	1.35 billion (2018)	412.7% of US
GDP	$2.73 trillion (2018)	13.3% of US
Land Area	1.27 million sq mi	32% of US

though it is considering a national bill to rectify some of the gaps between regions.

Bottlenecks and lack of access to public healthcare facilities have led to private insurance and non-public medical facilities offering services at drastically increased costs, more akin to the American private insurance system than actual universal healthcare; but with far less in quality and safety standards due to a lack of licensing and monitoring systems.

Should the crisis in healthcare continue in the United States, our nation will face similar systemic healthcare issues. Urban locales will end up with abundant, affordable healthcare while rural areas suffer a dearth of accessibility and affordability. Both the Medicaid and Medicare systems attempt to mitigate the coverage challenge, but are not as successful when it comes to the accessibility dilemma and the limitations of telemedicine. Should anything happen to these two systems, our nation will begin to look more like the two nations above than any previously reviewed nations thus far.

As is evidenced, all of the reviewed nations (except China and India) benefit from the concept of *fettered capitalism;* that government regulation is needed to control healthcare costs and ensure affordable coverage for everyone. From relegating direct control of all aspects of national healthcare to funding and delegating control to regional governments, it should be noted that few of the nations reviewed cover everything at 100%. In fact, cost sharing, even with the closest thing to single-payer (the UK), still exists as a necessary financial mechanism on top of taxes and other funding.

The native users of these programs are not without their lists of problems, complaints, and issues with their healthcare system. **They will also openly and loudly admit that it is leagues superior and preferable to the system of the United States.** They can't believe that in America healthcare isn't a *right* but a privilege only for those able to afford it, much less that we aren't making any attempts to fix it. They applauded half-heartedly at the passing of the ACA, but still think of our healthcare system as stuck in the Dark Ages.

Unfortunately what they, and the majority of Americans, don't understand is that while there is a vocal outcry to change healthcare for the better, there are rather large roadblocks both in infrastructure and society needing to be recognized and addressed first.

Nation*	US	CA	AU	UK	FR	DE	IT	JP	ES
Population (millions)	*327.1*	37.1	24.9	66.4	65	83.1	60.6	127.2	46.7
GDP (trillions)	*$20.5*	$1.71	$1.43	$2.83	$2.78	$4.01	$2.07	$4.97	$1.43
Land Area (million sq mi)	*3.797*	3.855	2.970	0.094	0.249	0.138	0.116	0.146	0.195
Universal Healthcare	*No*	Yes	Yes	Yes	Yes	Yes	Yes	Yes	Yes
Federal Funding	*Yes*	Yes	Yes	Yes	Yes	No	Yes	Yes	Yes
Regional Funding	*Yes*	Yes	Yes	No	No	Yes	Yes	No	Yes
Federal Regulation	*No*	Yes	Yes	Yes	Yes	Yes	Yes	Yes	Yes
Regional Regulation	*No*	Yes	Yes	No	No	No	Yes	No	Yes
Automatic Enrollment	*No*	Yes	Yes	Yes	Yes	No	Yes	No	Yes
Dental/Vision Coverage	*No*	No	No	Yes	No	No	No	Yes	No
Long-Term Care Coverage	*No*	No	No	Yes	Yes	No	No	Yes	No
Medical Out of Pocket Cost	*Yes*	No	Yes	No	Yes	Yes	Yes	Yes	Yes
Prescription Out of Pocket Cost	*Yes*	Yes	Yes	Yes	Yes	Yes	Yes	Yes	Yes
Insurance Available	*Yes*	Yes	Yes	Yes	Yes	Yes	Yes	Yes	Yes

*US-United States; CA-Canada; AU-Australia; UK-United Kingdom; FR-France; DE-Germany; IT-Italy; JP-Japan; ES-Spain

AMERICAN "ISSUES"

Though mine is not a popular opinion amongst my peers, progressives, or some of the Democratic Party, I'm afraid that single-payer healthcare is not a policy we should put forth at this time. As I stated, single-payer is aspirational, an ideal. It's something to strive for, but it's not necessarily the best solution for our nation at present. Instead, we should be striving for universal healthcare - one that works within the system we now have to *change* it for the better, and takes us towards that ideal of single-payer.

The reason it's important to work with the system is that, unlike other nations, the United States healthcare industry is, at its foundation, *not* a medical care delivery industry. **It's a jobs program.** It's unintentionally become a major component shoring up the economy and providing income and stability for people. As a benefit and byproduct it provides health and treatment for the citizens of the nation.

There are structural, political, and cultural realities today that must be acknowledged. These are more than simple roadblocks on the path to universal healthcare; they are national issues to be addressed, and not just in healthcare.

Federal Healthcare Systems

The woes and issues with commercial insurance and for-profit healthcare in our nation are extensive and well-known to everyone in America. However,

Population	327.1 million (2018)
GDP	$20.5 trillion (2018)
Land Area	3.797 million sq mi

lesser known is the fact that there are four federal healthcare programs run by the government: the Veterans Administration (VA), Tricare, Medicare, and Medicaid. This is the United States' form of government healthcare; but thanks to free market capitalism and its lack of *fettered capitalism*, they are not nearly as regulated as their international counterparts. As a result, they suffer from issues that provide less coverage and much higher costs for American denizens.

Veterans Administration (VA)

The non-active duty and retired military personnel healthcare system is a successful example of a single-payer system in the nation. The Federal government negotiates directly with pharmaceutical companies, manufacturers, and sets reimbursement rates; then funds everything directly through taxpayer expenses and administered through federal agencies throughout the nation. This is the closest thing to the UK's NHS we have, and the recent expansion to allow doctors outside the VA to treat patients and be reimbursed for it is a huge step in ensuring coverage for all members.

It should be noted however, the VA is not funded through the defense budget, and, due to political sabotage in the form of almost continual budget cuts for the last forty years, it now suffers personnel deficiencies and occasional treatment delays. Pharmaceutical companies make no secret of going along with this system only due to its small market share and potential bad press by not participating. The move to increase privatization incrementally toward full privatization is proposed constantly by the political party most enamored by the free markets.

Tricare

Closely related to the VA, this is the healthcare system for military personnel and their dependents. This program *is* funded by the Department of Defense (DoD), unlike the VA, and provides medical, dental, and vision healthcare to its members. Its drug formulary is rather large, and already includes options for patients to see doctors outside its system. Though many think Tricare is like the VA - run and administered by the government - it is not.

The US government and DoD in particular have contracted out the administration to two for-profit institutions in 2018, divided by region:

- Tricare West, run by Health Net, covering everything north and west of Oklahoma
- Tricare East, run by Humana, covering everything east of the Mississippi and the southern states including Texas

These companies are responsible for customer service, setting coverage policies, and reimbursement rates. Ultimately, these decisions are approved by the DoD Military Health System; but nonetheless, these for-profit institutions are responsible for healthcare administration. A third for-profit institution, Blue Cross Blue Shield of South Carolina, is contracted to process all the claims for both insurance companies in an effort to reduce administrative costs.

In fairness, few who benefit from the Tricare system complain of the coverage. In fact, all but one plan of Tricare (Tricare Prime, the HMO) rate quality, cost, and access to care at 85% (Tricare Prime was at 60%); though this has been declining since the reduced plan options of 2018. Still, this healthcare service designed to benefit active military members and their families has taxpayer money going to for-profit companies with little to no accountability of how the money is spent.

Medicare

This is the system everyone likes to quote ("Medicare for All"), but few understand how it works. To begin with, the only 100% coverage is for hospital inpatient stays, called Part A Medicare. Part B Medicare, which must be voluntarily enrolled in, covers only 80% of healthcare costs outside of the hospital once an annual deductible is met, not counting prescriptions, vision, or dental. Recently-implemented Part D prescription plan is another voluntary enrollment option which covers prescriptions, but at varying costs depending on the drug and the plan.

None of these plans are "free" to citizens of the United States. As of 2016, Part A now has an annual deductible before covering 100% and there are limitations to the number of days before patients must start paying for their in hospital stay. Part B also has an annual deductible, and the cost of the coverage gap is often dealt with by a Medicare Supplement (or MediGap) plan, run by for-profit insurance companies at a monthly cost. Part D not only has copay and deductible costs, but also a "donut hole" where patients are responsible for 100% of the cost of their drugs until they meet a specific out-of-pocket amount. This full-price donut hole was specially negotiated during the implementation of the Part D program by the pharmaceutical companies. The ACA is "closing" that donut hole, however it is being replaced with a flat 25% coinsurance payment for all medications after the plan deductible and until patients meet their out-of-pocket limit.

Medicare also offers to cover one vision check per year, though not lenses or glasses, and no dental. People can turn to separate insurance policies, or opt for a Part C plan, which cover everything from Part A, B, occasionally D, and sometimes more. This is done through private insurance companies that administer the plan, and can make minor changes, such as adding authorization gateways, some limitations on drug options, and adding their own network of doctors.

Most importantly, this program is not actually implemented and administered by the federal government, but contracted out to private for-profit entities. The federal government creates national advisory criteria that are baseline standards that need to be met; and then local, multi-state administrators set their guidelines and reimbursement prices based on these national guidelines. This does offer some pricing and cost limitations; but as more and more people opt for private insurance over public - one-third (33%) of all Medicare beneficiaries opted for Part C coverage in 2017 - it is likely that, as with the 2016 decision for a Part A deductible, additional costs to the patients will be implemented.

Medicaid
The program which some people are aware of, many politicize, and few understand. Medicaid is a healthcare

program set up state-by-state to provide coverage to those with low resources and limited income. It is partially-funded by the state and partially-funded by the federal government, and includes the Children's Healthcare Insurance Program (CHIP) to ensure children of limited income aren't without healthcare.

Coverage, eligibility, and enrollment requirements are determined by the states themselves. In states like California, Washington, and New York, not only did they accept an expansion proposal by the Affordable Care Act (ACA) to ensure more people were covered by healthcare, their coverage is expansive and sometimes more comprehensive than other government plans (like the VA). However, other states such as Texas, Alabama, and Wisconsin have limited not only coverage, at times they limit the ability to enroll or remain in the program by instituting an enrollment lottery, work requirements, and copays. This state-by-state patchwork variation of healthcare coverage is perhaps the best map of how divisive the concept of healthcare is in this nation.

Once again, the state governments rarely directly administer their plans. Administration contracts go to "middlemen" and result in an increased cost of care. In fact, the majority (80%) of Medicaid recipients are actually enrolled in managed care organizations (MCO). These are private, for-profit insurance companies contracted by the states to run the Medicaid programs. These, by law, must provide low costs (and low reimbursement) for healthcare treatments; but, as a result, many of these have created limited networks of providers that create long wait times and preferential treatment for non-Medicaid patients. It should be noted, however, that with the exception of delays, it has *not* typically resulted in a lower standard of care for the patients.

As you can see from the four programs above, the United States has approached crossing the line into *fettered capitalism*, especially with the VA. The ACA also introduced value-based payments for Medicare versus fee-for-service; that is, payments based on the *quality* and success of healthcare services rather than the *quantity* of services provided. While some studies have shown that contracting out has led to a savings in healthcare costs, it means income taxes are being directly funneled to for-profit, private industry in the billions of dollars. The number of jobs through these companies is, of course, good for the economy as a whole; but does it offset the for-profit model that other nations have "fettered" with similar - some would say, superior, care outcome results? And since these companies and the national workforce are so intricately linked with healthcare, how can we make wholesale changes that won't cause irreparable harm to the nation in the process?

Controversial Coverage: Diverse Opinions of a Diverse Nation

When I consider the challenges for a national single-payer or universal healthcare plan, the immediate issue that springs to mind is the question: can the citizens of the United States, nationally or regionally, agree on what needs to be covered by national healthcare insurance? In order to implement national universal healthcare controversial healthcare treatments must be settled almost uniformly across the nation. Though there are far too many to address in this quick narrative, some of the most easily visible issues are:

Reproductive Issues

The Hyde Amendment currently on federal law books states that federal funds can't be used for abortions except in extreme circumstances. That being said, if a disabled woman on Medicare got pregnant and decided to terminate the pregnancy, it is technically fully covered by Medicare guidelines as a medical procedure; it's just not reimbursable.

I, and I'm sure many of you reading this, can easily imagine the conservative clergymen and politicians standing up and objecting to allowing federal funds pay for abortions and birth control despite the hypocrisy of these same groups insisting federal funds pay for vasectomies and Viagra. Religious institutions would ask for waivers to avoid paying for such procedures, followed quickly by corporations and then states.

The Federal government, if they granted the waivers, would immediately doom universal coverage because it would no longer be universal, but a return to a patchwork system. California, for instance, would cover all contraceptive options. Texas might have a city or two, but much of the state would demand a waiver. If the government instead denies the waivers, these same groups would cry out about dictatorships and abuse of power.

In 2017, 40% of the nation, regardless of religious and political affiliation, currently agree that contraception (and specifically abortion) should be illegal according to the Pew Research Center. Until that number is down to, at most 10%, that large minority objection will continue to derail any attempt at national coverage.

Vaccines

The Anti-Vaccine movement (anti-vaxxers) has gained enough steam over the last half decade that near-extinct diseases like the measles have made a resurgence, as in Minnesota and California. Despite being a minority opinion in the nation and scientific world, both left and right-leaning families are a part of this movement with devastating results to their local communities.

Instituting single-payer or universal healthcare would include policies and procedures that mandate minimizing exposure to preventable diseases, and end this increasingly vocal minority. Instead of the patchwork state system where some people can reject vaccine treatments on philosophical or religious grounds, the nation would instead follow California, West Virginia, and Mississippi and allow exemptions only on extreme medical grounds.

To allow exemptions would not only endanger the greater population but invite additional exemptions. For instance, if parents have a religious exemption to vaccines, why would they pay taxes to support *others* getting vaccines in a single-payer system? If they have a philosophical objection to non-holistic treatments, why are they paying taxes to support a medical industry that primarily uses it? In our litigious nation these sound like outlandish scenarios but would undoubtedly come to pass.

We already see such complications and objections today by Jehovah's Witnesses who need waivers for blood transfusions, while Christian Scientists don't believe in modern medicine or medical treatment. Under universal healthcare not only would they have to pay for the services whether used or not, but also their children (and maybe themselves) would be required to accept vaccines for the good of the nation. Penalties for not vaccinating would likely mimic other nations, such as withholding government benefits, harsh financial fines for the parents, and even being charged with child endangerment.

Until these issues are resolved via an "exemption clause" treatment set-up for these groups, or an executive, legislative, or judicial decision that these organizations must accept and take part of the system with no appeal option, this is yet another complication to instituting national healthcare.

Mental Health

Mental health is very much a gray area throughout the nation. Even though diagnoses like depression, bipolar disorder, and attention deficit are real, treatable, and recognized; there are an equal number of people who don't believe in therapy, medication, or even the diseases themselves. There are many who would tell the mentally ill to "get more God in their life," to "interact with more people," and to "get off the drugs and eat healthy." And while some of these suggestions offer some benefit; it also disregards the complexity and difficulty of living with and treating mental illness.

It's not just public opinion, either. Both the federal government and private sectors cover mental health at a reduced rate. There's lower reimbursement for services, lower coverage for treatment, and more limited networks for doctors to treat such disorders. While some states and the ACA are attempting to change this disparity into equality, it's still a 5-10 year plan and not everyone is following suit or focusing on this necessity, and Medicare and Medicaid are currently exempt from this transition.

In developing a universal healthcare situation, can we as a nation agree that depression is a medical disorder? And while recently these issues have become more visible in the public eye, there is still a social stigma attached that means there will be a significant number of objections to people paying for this segment of our society.

Substance Abuse

Are drug users criminals or patients? Can an addict seek medical treatment or is it better to let them go cold turkey in a cell? What about alcoholics, where do they stand? Should AA be covered by health care? Should the unhealthy side-effects of a lifelong smoker get medical treatment; or like the addict, should they suffer for poisoning their own body?

These are questions from the political right *and* left, and no two people have the same answer. Should marijuana be legalized and regulated? Or should it only be for medicinal use? Or is it too dangerous to allow as a treatment at all? Should attempts to stop smoking be covered by insurance, or should the person cover the costs themselves, or should the tobacco industry pay for the treatment?

Much like contraception and mental health, the debate has raged for decades and, again, there needs to be a national, or at least regional, majority agreement within the nation. Like mental health these issues have become more and more visible recently; but any national plan would have to address these questions and be prepared to defend their position. Unfortunately this is often left as a grey area to address while planning a national healthcare proposal in more specific detail.

These examples all show that, bottom line, we need to have a national discussion on these issues - among myriad others - before we can ever consider a universal healthcare policy, much less the ideal of single-payer. Should a Democratic unified federal government in 2021 institute a national healthcare plan, they would have to construct a Constitutional way to prevent governors and various special interest groups from objecting or blocking coverage through the courts to avoid a similar issue like the incongruous Medicaid Expansion for the ACA.

      Unfortunately, there isn't an easy soundbite. How do you condense this issue to five minutes, much less five words, that can be easily ingested and understood by the nation? My condensed examples here take pages and don't address all the details and complications that could arise. It is a sad fact that any national healthcare system is doomed until we, as a nation, finally come to a consensus (or at least a large majority) on these and many other issues.

Negative Economic Impact

Pundits, politicians, and activists often like to quote that healthcare spending is nearly 20% of the United States GDP, and most likely will reach that exact percentage by 2025. That's approximately one-fifth of our economy that current single-payer proposals are aimed at redesigning. Even on a smaller scale - California, for instance - healthcare GDP was also at 18% in 2015. To put this into perspective, one-fifth of the nation's economy employs approximately 20 million people. Not just doctors, but researchers, medical secretaries, psychologists, biomedical engineers, and dozens more occupations identified by the US Census bureau.

Those are the easily identifiable medical occupations. There are also statisticians, janitors, transportation specialists, sales, marketing, and a myriad of other jobs ancillary to the healthcare industry. At a low-ball estimate with these additional professions, 25 million people are employed by, or their employment is directly linked to, the US healthcare industry and economy. Which, unsurprisingly, is also 20% of all employed individuals in the nation. And a single-payer transition will affect all of them, most in a negative way.

For argument's sake, let's say all doctors and nurses will remain employed, meaning approximately 11 million people will be unaffected. Removing the ancillary jobs, that leaves 9 million who likely face disruption. To reduce administrative costs, every person employed by an insurance company, from the board of directors to middle management to the answering service will be evaluated and, most likely, dismissed. The government will take on some of the employees, but with no competing insurance companies, a medical office doesn't need to employ three people to verify insurance, work through authorizations, and handle claims.

Given the government model, all billing will eventually be transitioned to a uniform format.

Outside the physician's office potentially half of all sales representatives from various drug companies will be immediately laid off, as there will no longer need to be in contact with the offices or to compete with each other for patients. The pharmaceutical companies will have their lobbyists and consultants already in touch with the federal government to do that job. Patient specialists who assisted in getting funding and drugs for those unable to afford treatment would likewise be let go as the government plan guarantees not only access to the drug but affordability. Medical manufacturers will also suffer, as the government law requiring the lowest bid means those with plants outside the US will be able to lowball domestic manufacturers. Alternatively, domestic manufacturers will need to return manufacturing to US shores and citizens may have to be willing to pay higher costs for healthcare.

At the most optimistic, with government hiring many in-office and corporate support staff, maybe 50%, around 4.5 million people, will be gainfully employed after a conversion to single-payer. Again, this assumes no doctors or nurses get laid off, or depart due to the reimbursement rate or patient demands. These are not unskilled jobs, and with the removal of such a large segment of the economy, there will be an influx of skilled labor and a lack of employment opportunities in external industries as many will have had careers in healthcare that don't translate beyond low-paying jobs. This would create not only a large disgruntled segment of the population, but an explosion of the unemployment rate.

For the 5 million ancillary jobs, some results can be predicted. The transportation industry will be contracted to only a select few companies, and most likely to those already working with the government. Nonprofits who have built their existence on helping those with financial healthcare issues will have to find another cause or dissolve entirely. Those employed by the paper industry to create forms in triplicate and write contracts for each insurance and hospital cooperative will be downsized dramatically. And janitorial staff will find themselves replaced with government-approved contractors. Again, being optimistic, perhaps 1 million of the jobs will survive the transition to single-payer.

Finally, there's the small-business start-up industry. Healthcare in general has had a recent explosion of small businesses develop from new treatments, new testing methods, even new software development. A transition to single-payer will put a significant, maybe insurmountable, damper on these small industries. Unless sanctioned by the national single-payer system, these industries would find no market to reach. Instead, they would have to go through the process of not only contracting with the federal government, but integrating their new product - some untested - into the national system. And without data, such as long-term use, or proof of increased efficacy, or even business need, these small businesses will cease to exist, exterminating an entire segment of consulting and innovating industry that America has prided itself on for over a century.

While the estimation of potential small-businesses is impossible to predict, given the numbers above a single-payer transition will, at best, result in 8.5 million people displaced from their jobs. To put that into perspective, the unemployment rate as of 2019 is approximately 3.6%, or 5.8 million people. A single-payer transition, even phased in over a number of years, could potentially triple the unemployment rate to 9.8%, or 14.3 million unemployed persons. Granted, some of the single-payer plans, H.R.676 especially, includes provisions to hire from the healthcare industry first, pay for retraining, and provide the missing salary for 2 years, with no contingency if it takes longer to reintegrate the workforce elsewhere in the economy. Even with that, to replace the complex, intricate healthcare industry we have now with a single-payer system will lead to a steep short-term economic fall, and possibly a depression the likes of which we've not seen since 1929. It's a massive social engineering task to repurpose not just an industry, but millions of workers.

A universal healthcare system not designed around single-payer should lessen the economic impact, potentially saving jobs and having only a marginal unemployment boost. When examining how to transform nearly 20% of the nation's economy, we have to keep in mind that *any* change can affect any of these sectors, and must brace and prepare for it accordingly. There will be fallout in the above economic sectors, to how much and what degree will depend on how diligent and thorough the potential healthcare legislation will be.

National Mindset

When travelling the world, many people in countries with universal healthcare: Canada, the U.K., Germany, Australia, can't fathom how in the United States healthcare is a privilege, not a right. Those same international policies occasionally penalize tourists of those countries for using healthcare in the U.S. because of the high cost that can be incurred. International citizens find themselves shocked that a U.S. ambulance ride, free or low-cost in their own nation, is a $400 bill that their national insurance will pass on to them.

In the U.S. itself, however, few people from any political leanings believe that universal healthcare is a right or are willing to pay for it beyond themselves. During the 2016 election Vox News media surveyed American voters on if they were willing to pay higher taxes for healthcare. An average of 70% of Democratic voters were willing to pay compared to only 40% of Republican voters. Yet when asked specifics, hard numbers or a percentage, a two-thirds majority of *Democratic* voters in 2015 were unwilling to pay more than $1000 yearly for national insurance. The average family of four insurance premium (cost) for a year of healthcare in 2015 was $5000.

In fairness, some Democrats did the math and determined they would save money with higher taxes when healthcare costs were not a concern. Nonetheless, this survey reveals that even within the most progressive aspects of our nation there is a reluctance to share the burden of cost in an effort to uplift the quality of life for everyone. To quote Vox, "they don't want to Feel the Bern in their wallets." In fact, in a recent 2017 survey, the Kaiser Family Foundation (KFF) found 53% national support for a government-run health plan across the political spectrum, but that support dropped once higher taxes are introduced as a way to pay for it.

This mindset is half of the problem. The other half is that we, as Americans, don't view healthcare as a right. Atul Gawande wrote in <u>The New Yorker</u> that he returned to his hometown in Ohio to ask about universal healthcare. He discovered that people wanted health care for themselves, but were unwilling to pay to cover someone else. This can be traced all the way back to "the welfare queen myth," that certain people are lazy or unmotivated, so why should they reap the benefits of another's hard work?

It's an issue that permeates our society since our first settlers. From property rights to food stamps to college education, we have wrestled with what is the government's duty in regards to helping the disadvantaged, injured, or ill; and how much responsibility (fiscal or otherwise) each person should contribute to the solution. Again, go to other nations and the same set of debates exists, except not with healthcare. In healthcare, they are all equal because they all contribute, and so they all reap the benefits.

Whether this is a cultural mindset, a result of recovery from World Wars, or even a political party taking unilateral action, the people of these nations have agreed collectively about how healthcare should be handled in their country. The closest America has ever been united on a national decision was after the bombing of Pearl Harbor when we stood together to enter World War II. Even 9/11 did not unify us as effectively. As the schisms between political and socioeconomic groups grow, it is less likely we can have a cogent, cohesive, coherent conversation on where we want to go regarding national healthcare.

Financial Viability

I'm sure you've all been waiting for this most popular argument regarding single-payer or universal healthcare. So let me be explicitly clear and say that the inability to institute single-payer or universal healthcare due to the cost or financial burden is, without a doubt, ***not*** a reason national healthcare won't happen. Not only does Medicare and the Veterans Admin (VA) function based on federal taxes and price control, but dozens of other nations around the world have proven this is a false argument to present when trying to end the universal healthcare debate.

The fact is the financial argument against universal healthcare is essentially moot. When you have a large enough economy and the population to support it, universal healthcare is one of the most efficient, effective methods of national healthcare reform. While Vermont and Colorado struggled to meet this metric, California with its economy of scale *could* implement it. And if the 6th largest economy of the world could hypothetically do it (along with all the smaller economies of the world), so can the 1st.

Every politician and newscaster will cite cost as the primary reason universal healthcare is not viable because it's a simple soundbite, especially when riling up small government and conservative constituents. There are other controversial and complicated reasons national healthcare reform isn't viable at this time, as listed above. However the actual financial cost, the price tag, is not a valid one.

That's not to say financial viability hasn't been a roadblock for attempts in the United States before. Vermont tried to institute single-payer and failed citing the cost of the program. Healthy California, California's single-payer initiative, was shelved specifically because of the high cost and lack of funding incorporated into the bill. Even Senator Sanders' Medicare for All bill, S.915, faces the financial viability challenge as, like California, it doesn't include funding directly in the bill and will, according to its critics, explode the deficit.

It's true the cost of a national universal healthcare bill is incalculable, not because health is unpredictable or because some events (i.e., natural disasters) are unforeseen. Cost is incalculable because the negotiations that would take place to set prices on procedures, medications, and physician salaries aren't proposed in any bill, but set to be negotiated during implementation. On a national level, there would also be regional pricing on salaries and facility reimbursement simply based on population density and demand for services.

In addition, there's the change in personal and business income due to taxation. Even with tax rates set and known for both parties, the estimated cost per person is again, only an estimate. Each person will save by not having to pay for their personal care; but each person's current cost for healthcare varies from company to company, from age to region, from insurance company to medical co-op. Businesses large and small could be facing an increase or decrease depending on the plan, their size, and their gross income. It's extremely volatile and no one, particularly politicians, wants to get into the complexities of raising taxes, even for a good cause.

None of the above is a reason why national healthcare reform isn't financially viable for the United States. Yes, tax increases and income fluctuations will be as volatile as the stock market, and incomplete price negotiations are, unsurprisingly, an unknown factor. The truth is that none of it actually matters. In terms of gross domestic product

(GDP), the United States is the 1st largest economy in the world, and California is the 6th. That's two domestic economies with a combined $20 trillion GDP (in 2015) to apply to the nation annually. Factor in that price control will feature heavily in a national healthcare plan, even the "outrageous" price of $4.9 trillion (the estimated cost of S.915) in annual health care costs is well within our capabilities as a nation. It's only one-fifth of our economy, the same as today.

The above details are, of course, not all-encompassing nor definitive on this topic. It may be that in the next five to ten years we as a country will have a national conversation; that we will define healthcare as a right and not a privilege, that controversies of vaccines and mental health can be settled, that the economy and jobs can survive with the right tools and policies in place. It's not impossible.

Just highly improbable.

To reiterate, I'm not saying single-payer healthcare is terrible or completely impossible. It's a fantastic ideal, a goal for us as a nation to strive for. We must remember that we can't turn this nation on a soundbite, and there's very real consequences that are not being considered or addressed by supporters, politicians, or pundits.

Just because other nations have it does not mean it's the best course for our nation. At least, not yet. While we're on the road to universal healthcare, however, we need to avoid easy pitfalls. "Medicare for All" is both a noble attempt and a meaningless slogan, a way to rile up people with little understanding of the complexities that would be involved in a significant change of one-fifth of our economy.

If we truly want to work towards a future of universal coverage, while we're helping evolve opinion and change attitudes, we need to introduce policies and ideas towards that future. Rome wasn't built in a day. **We have the advantage of a foundation both in Medicare and the Affordable Care Act. Neither are perfect, but with a policy change here, a regulation proposal there, we can get to universal healthcare for all.**

IMPROVEMENT INITIATIVES:

BETTER HEALTHCARE NOW

From the previous sections we now can say single-payer isn't quite how the world handles healthcare, nor is universal healthcare going to be easy given the social and political situation in America. Nonetheless, there are things we *can* do or at least attempt to improve healthcare now. Maybe not today, but tomorrow and for generations to come. The following are suggestions for states to build towards better healthcare coverage, maybe even pave the way to national universal healthcare.

I say 'states' because currently the national level is not viable to implement any of the following suggestions. Not only would it require a discussion and consensus our current mindsets aren't willing to tackle, but the challenge from right-leaning political states would endanger or even destroy proposals at the courts, much as they did with the Medicaid Expansion in the ACA. As Europe shows, states with smaller populations and surface area but high GDP can successfully implement universal healthcare directives, with the hope that such examples would lead to national reform.

The following proposals will be presented as tiers of changing, each level building on proposals from the previous tier. Some of the proposals are drawn from the international models reviewed, some are taken from single-payer legislation that have been proposed already, and some will be my own ideas based on observations and interactions after a decade in the healthcare industry. Ideally, each tier would be implemented uniformly and built up over time to create increased coverage with more efficient and cost effective healthcare for everyone.

That being said, I deliberately present these as *individual* initiative proposals because, as we've seen with previous attempts across the nation, when just one section is unpopular or can't be implemented, the entire attempt at healthcare reform collapses. In this way legislators can propose each initiative on its own and have it stand on its own merit, rather than as part of an enormous and perhaps unfathomable reform.

It is also why I have relegated financial suggestions for funding these initiatives to its own section at the end. Some states, such as Colorado and California, have written into law that marijuana sales must support healthcare initiatives, so funding for some lower-cost proposals is already available for those states. Other states, such as Texas, could follow Alaska's example and create an additional tax on natural resource companies. While some proposals will require larger financial resources than others, and may need entire tax overhauls, others states may be able to institute them with existing systems. I leave it to the tax experts and legislatures to determine which financial proposals work best for which state to implement their own healthcare reforms.

Tier One

These initiative proposals are the simplest of improvements states can make to improve their healthcare systems. Some of these states have already implemented, others are pulled directly from healthcare reform proposals currently in legislative limbo. These, more than any other tier, have little to no cost for the states themselves, and are the foundations of better healthcare for all.

Affordable Care Act

This seems almost ridiculous to add, but as some states have shown, even federal law is not above ignoring. As a few have already done, states should enshrine the ACA insurance guidelines as state laws *to reinforce* federal law. This means no exclusion for pre-existing situations, no gender-based pricing, no maximum limitations and out-of-pocket cost limiters to name just a few benefits. As long as the federal law is threatened by even a minority, it's up to the states to reinforce a program that a majority of the US population has deemed worthy of their support in regards to its continuance.

Mandatory Coverage

Both 'Medicare for All' bills in Congress and 'Healthy California' expanded what healthcare services must be covered by insurances. Of the three, Healthy California was the most comprehensive, including emergency transportation (ambulances), hospice care, substance abuse treatment, podiatric care, chiropractic care, all vaccines, acupuncture, rehabilitative and habilitative services. On a state level, the Department of Insurance can issue an edict that all insurance coverage in the state must cover these aspects in addition to medical, dental, vision and mental health treatment. That insurance won't cover the ambulance ride in an emergency is outrageous, forcing you to spend your savings to save your life. Everything will be argued against by insurance companies; but the precedent is already set in terms of mandatory minimums for insurance coverage thanks to the ACA.

Health Reimbursement Parity
Although some states are already attempting to implement this, a number have not instituted reimbursement parity-equal coverage - for mental and physical health. Many insurance plans either don't cover, or cover minimally, mental health. One plan, for instance, may have treatments for everything from cancer to whooping cough be covered at 80%; but that same plan covers mental health coverage from depression to schizophrenia at only 45%. This is one reason behavioral health can be more expensive than medical care and equalizing it so everything from depression to cancer is covered at the same rate is a minor, but important, nuance to help keep a growing aspect of healthcare accessibility available.

Another parity issue comes from dental and vision coverage. For instance many if not all dental plans have a maximum cap. After this amount (usually $1,000 - $3,000) the patient is responsible for all costs associated with dental work. For those with orthodontic costs (mostly the young) and implants and appliances (mostly the elderly) this can be prohibitively expensive. The ACA instituted out-of-pocket maximums to ensure those with lots of healthcare issues weren't priced out of seeking treatment. This has not yet been applied to dental or vision insurance and should be. An easy idea to resolve this issue would be to apply dental and vision costs towards the annual medical out-of-pocket maximum (on average $6000).

Though both dental and vision industries would disagree, much like physical and mental health, there shouldn't be a financial limit that precludes people from seeking treatment. Once again, the states can institute a directive detailing that both dental and vision insurances cannot have a maximum cap - mirroring the ACA healthcare guidelines. That may result in different coverage state-to-state, but dental hygiene and ability to see are important, essential, and can reduce medical costs while vastly improving quality of life.

Upfront Payment
An unsettling trend across the nation is for hospitals and other healthcare facilities to insist on payment up front rather than post-procedure, including people with insurance that would cover said procedures. Due to hospitals being wary of insurances deciding *not* to cover a procedure at the last minute, they are insisting patients pay the full cost upfront, occasionally offering financing options and private, sometimes predatory loans.

This is akin to the problem that used to plague emergency rooms, where patients without insurance would arrive and not be treated simply because the hospital wouldn't be reimbursed for the treatment. It was better to not treat the patient at all than take a financial loss. It wasn't until the federal government passed a law mandating hospital ERs *must* stabilize all patients and states could work out reimbursement or face financial liability for non-treatment that the issue got somewhat resolved. To this day there are stories of those with insurance getting preferential treatment, but that can only be addressed as the stories come out or until states begin more stringent audits of hospital activities. There are some investigating these issues, such as reporter Sarah Kiff at Vox Media who has been investigating ER costs and responses.

However, this proposal could work on the state level, since the federal government isn't going to make any adjustments soon. In this case, states can mandate that, like diners or hotels or haircuts, no upfront cost can be demanded or required for patients until the service and/or treatment is performed. The *only* exception would be copays, which are often collected upon entering a physician's office or for non-emergent patients in ERs, but even that could be changed into a post-visit payment.

Without this regulation, patients with less financial means will be penalized and suffer more health complications than those with better insurance and greater income. If we want to create uniform treatment of all patients, this must be instituted.

Tier Two

While the above are simply States updating legislation and definitions for coverage and reimbursement, the next proposals, while not overly complicated, are slightly more difficult to implement. All of these proposals are tied in with State Medicaids, and include potentially transforming the systems in place. Some of these will not be viable for every State, and some will be painful financially; but there's enough flexibility in the proposals below that many states should be able to implement at least some of the suggestions below.

Expanded Medicaid Coverage

This is not in reference to the ACA's Medicaid Expansion program. Instead, this is similar to the *Mandatory Coverage* initiative in Tier One, except for State Medicaids. In California, Medicaid covers not only physical health, but mental health, dental, vision, and prescriptions. Not every state has such generous Medicaid coverage, even though vision and dental are just as crucial to health. This initiative is simple: mandate that State Medicaid *cover* the additional programs. It may seem like this isn't needed, but in July 2018 Kentucky attempted to cut both dental and vision from its Medicaid program. Rather than leave the coverage at the mercy of political whims or fiscal policy, this would ensure the coverage is always there.

Medicaid Fund Integration

Medicaid is funded from two sources: state taxes and the federal government. However, there are at least two Medicaid funds: one for Medicaid, and one for the Children's Health Insurance Program (CHIP), which ensures all children, regardless of economic circumstance, get healthcare coverage.

Some states, however, have merged these funds together into a combined state fund. Rather than have two state funds, two programs to administer and track, it's more cost-effective to put all the financing together. States would still need administrators to track recipients and audit both programs, but they could reduce administrative costs by removing the oversight of an entire fund via consolidation. For states with separate Social Security and Disability (SS and SSDI) Medicaid funds, the same cost-savings from CHIP could apply to their programs as well by merging all their financing into the main Medicaid fund.

The downside of this proposal is that it may require permission from the Federal Government to implement. However, this waiver has been issued multiple times before with highly successful results, both before and after the ACA was implemented. In the interest of balancing state budgets and streamlining funding programs for Medicaid to all parties, there's no reason besides politics for a denial to be forthcoming, nor for states to not pursue such an initiative.

Mandatory Medicaid Licensing
One of the most difficult issues facing states today is the lack of physicians enrolled in the Medicaid programs. Doctors don't have to accept Medicaid patients; they volunteer into the state program and its network. Thanks to the low reimbursement rate, fewer and fewer doctors sign up to treat Medicaid patients. A controversial solution is, when applying for or renewing a State medical license, making Medicaid enrollment a mandatory aspect of obtaining said license.

This doesn't mean doctors are forced to see *only* Medicaid patients. If their practices are full, they can refuse to accept new patients (or any patients, for that matter). By making them required to accept Medicaid patients, a less busy office can't turn away patients simply because they don't like the reimbursement rates. This wouldn't just apply to physicians. Dentists, psychiatrists, any healthcare professional who gets a state license would be able to treat anyone in Medicaid.

Obviously, physicians would very strenuously argue against it, and it might even drive some out of practice, as was said when physician Medicare enrollment was first instituted. Much like that Medicare enrollment initiate, though, most would remain and make the adjustment. There are additional steps states can take to mitigate the push-back as well, such as increase Medicaid reimbursement (see below) or even offer additional benefits to being licensed in the state (see Tier Three).

Medicaid Reimbursement

Two reimbursement rates that physicians often complain about are Medicare and Medicaid. Medicaid is often drastically reduced compared to Medicare, and it's the primary reason physicians turn away Medicaid patients. There is a simple solution to this issue, though no States will actually like it because it will increase state healthcare costs. Still, if an increase in Medicaid physicians occurs, to help mitigate doctor frustrations and prevent poor treatment outcomes by seeing too many patients to make a profit, the simplest solution is to raise the Medicaid reimbursement rate (and uniform costs, see Tier Four).

This will be one of the most difficult proposals to pass based on the fact that it is a direct increase in healthcare costs for the state. Nonetheless it's something that must be addressed, *especially* if all doctors are mandated to see

Medicaid patients. Three potential solutions are (from most to least cost-effective):

- Increase the Medicaid reimbursement to an average of the Medicaid and Medicare rates
- Tie the Medicaid reimbursement to Medicare minus 6% (Medicare - 6%)
- Tie Medicaid reimbursement to Medicare plus 5% (Medicare +5%)

Doctors would most like the last one, obviously, the first one would make States happiest. The benefit of the last two of the above is that the reimbursement has little upkeep or pushback year-to-year. By tying it to the Medicare reimbursement rate, there's no need to worry about adjustments at a later date - it's tied directly to the Federal guidelines, and adjusts as necessary to the national need automatically. This would also include medications, dental and vision coverage. For services not covered by Medicare, States could default to the first bullet point, though perhaps that wouldn't be an issue after the tie to the Medicare rate is set.

Tier Three

It is in these proposals where we really begin the build off the previous initiative proposals, and introduce the next set of building blocks for improving healthcare coverage and accessibility across the board. These will almost certainly require independent funding from the Funding Initiatives section, simply because the State will be instituting new programs requiring oversight, employees, perhaps new legislation.

Data Collection

'Healthy California' had an entire subsection dedicated to the collection of data from the hospital industry. Taken directly from the legislation it would collect:

- Inpatient discharge data, including acuity and risk of mortality
- Emergency department and ambulatory surgery data, including charge data, length of stay, and patients' unit of observation
- Hospital annual financial data, including all of the following:
  - Community benefits by hospital in dollar value
  - Number of employees and classification by hospital unit
  - Number of hours worked by hospital unit
  - Employee wage information by job title and hospital unit
  - Number of registered nurses per staffed bed by hospital unit
  - Type and value of healthy information technology

- ○ Annual spending on health information technology, including purchases, upgrades, and maintenance
- Protected Health Information (PHI), including names, age, and demographic info would *not* be collected to prevent any aggregation of the data above

This would be compiled in a primary state database accessible by the public, with authorization to offer grants for research on the efficacy of these systems, and how to not only improve them, but make them more equal across different regions of the state. This is an *excellent* proposal, and one I wish they'd instituted independently. Granted, the private hospitals wouldn't want to participate; but it could be instituted with state and medical school affiliated hospitals to get a sense of healthcare status and results in hospitals, as well as track healthcare debt on a regional basis across entire States.

Medical School Scholarships
In the unimplemented legislation of 'Healthy California,' the State would offer to cover tuition and costs (though not housing) of medical school in exchange for working for the state. Granted, in the 'Healthy California' legislation, all doctors would work for the state, there was no timeline; nonetheless, this is an excellent concept and needs only a few tweaks. I would adjust the legislation to include coverage for medical school, books, and reasonable housing in exchange for five years working directly for the state plus an additional five years working *in* the state in a professional capacity. However, this financial scholarship and support would only apply to those pursuing a Nurse Practitioner (NP) and General Practitioner (GP) degree.

It takes, on average, four to ten years to earn either degree respectively, so repayment by working the same time in the state is not excessive. The limitation to GP and NP is because both are in the greatest demand nationwide as they typically earn less than specialists. By having the first five years be state-mandated, states can direct new GPs and NPs to areas currently underserviced by physicians, and it provides a basis for these new physicians to build up their own careers without excess pressure from the job market.

The only other physician education I would suggest benefit from this program are psychiatrists and psychiatric NPs. There's a high demand for behavioral health providers who can also prescribe medications, especially for Medicaid and Medicare patients—the stable patients, at least. As the first five years would mandate they work for the state, this could help fill that need.

Mandated Licensing Benefits
In Tier Two, I introduced the idea of *Mandated Medicaid Licensing* for all doctors that get registered with the state. I mentioned the idea of a benefit to offset some of the pushback. Here it is: I would recommend the creation of a state malpractice department. When signing up for licensing and Medicaid, as a bonus physicians also enroll in a low-cost state-run malpractice insurance program. That means the state would handle all malpractice lawsuits and doctors wouldn't have to pay such high out-of-pocket costs themselves for lawyers.

This has its own pluses and minuses. In California, for instance, the laws regarding malpractice suits are very strict and so the State's liability is lower than say, New Jersey, where there is no limit on financial restitution or deadline to file a lawsuit. Ironically, it's the doctors in states like New Jersey where they would most trade the option of seeing Medicaid patients for much lower malpractice premiums (currently up to $100,000 per year).

This proposal creates a new department and financial cost to the State itself, and no State likes adding additional costs to its budget. It could lead to new medical malpractice legislation across the nation, which also disrupts the healthcare industry. It also hinders, if not severely damages, one of the peripheral industries I mentioned early on; and for all the "ambulance chasing lawyer" stereotypes we as a society openly mock, this would put some of those very real people out of work possibly for good. This is one of those trade-offs we'd have to decide as a society: is it better to increase access to healthcare, or to maintain an economically thriving part of the adjacent legal industry?

Tier Four

Now we begin to get to some of the more transformative proposals. Insurance standards have been set, Medicaid has been upgraded, new systems have been implemented. With these out of the way, States can begin implementing more complex steps towards universal coverage. These will draw more from the international community, and focus not only on improving state insurance, but regulating private insurance as well.

Uniform Costs

With the information from **Tier Three** *Data Collection,* a State could setup a set of uniform costs for all procedures, drugs, and other healthcare costs for patients. It couldn't be the Medicaid amount; in fact, this would be ideally set at least fifteen percent above the Medicare amount as the maximum reimbursement level (Medicare + 15%). The State would then legislate that this fee schedule must be followed for all healthcare providers. Insurance and pharmaceutical companies could not charge in excess of these costs.

Identifying the fee schedule would be complicated. The ACA mandates outcome-based metrics for reimbursement; hospitals must aim therefore for long-term healthier patients, rather than charging per-procedure, patient, or swift discharge. It also requires bundling procedures for reduced cost; but it specifically doesn't define those bundles, as each patient has their own unique needs. Determining how to evaluate bundling and reimbursement with a fee for service would be difficult but not impossible. Germany's reimbursement model would be an excellent foundation.

While the procedures and medical equipment could be universal, physician reimbursement would have to be regionalized. For instance, a doctor in San Francisco, CA has a higher cost of living (CoL) and needs higher reimbursement than the doctor in Redding, CA, who has lower CoL. Then a mitigation or reward system needs to be setup to prevent physicians from moving out of low CoL areas aiming for higher returns. This regionalized reimbursement would be all-inclusive, affecting pharmacists, dentists, et al. along with physicians.

That's before we get to the insurance companies screaming about loss of profit, impinging on their free trade, and the devaluation of their shareholder value. Nonetheless, this has already been done by Maryland, and California is now investigating a similar initiative. If multiple states could not just survive the lawsuits, but *win* them, then this is perhaps the greatest method in curbing healthcare costs to patients and decreasing healthcare costs overall across the states *and* the nation.

State Patient Database

Though few other nations have a national patient database, taking a page from Canada's policy and having statewide patient databases would be a great boon to increasing efficacy and consistent treatment records for patients. This would require developing a compatible and portable electronic healthcare record system officially adopted by a state government and mandated for all hospitals, doctor's offices, pharmacies and other healthcare providers to be used.

This would also mean that insurance and pharmaceutical companies would have to have systems compatible with the mandated state system, which may simplify claim submission across multiple insurance companies and cost tracking for pharmaceuticals. This would also put many states in compliance with the federal electronic records requirement, which is currently being slowly instituted in some states. The difference is that the federal records requirement doesn't specify that electronic systems have to be compatible with each other, let alone the entire state or nation.

Once again, doctors and the healthcare industry would object; but once instituted one group (doctors) would be relived of multiple logins and different electronic systems. The system could also follow Australia's system, to allow physicians and patients to access and provide input to the system. However, like the malpractice trade-off for requiring physicians to enroll in Medicaid, there is a detriment to the electronic records industry. Programmers, sales reps, an entire industry would be locked out: once a state has mandated a system, others can still be used, but why would offices opt for more than one? The other option is to mandate all electronic record systems be compatible with each other and with a statewide patient database.

Transition to Nonprofits
One of the common themes through the international healthcare section is the governments often required healthcare industries to be or include not-for-profit institutions. This is something that should definitely be instituted on the national level. Failing that, states could require all contractors administering Medicaid programs to be nonprofit. Obviously, this couldn't happen overnight, and states can't force private companies to become nonprofits. They can, however, institute a five-year transition for all state healthcare contracts over to nonprofit entities. That gives time for private companies to either convert to nonprofit,

create nonprofit entities within their structures, or, if for-profit companies reject this, the five years allows nonprofit companies to form, set up, and begin contracting with the governments.

There would be minimal job loss, as those in the for-profit industry could transition to the nonprofit, either if the company changed or by being hired by new nonprofits. It encourages entrepreneurship and increases transparency thanks to the state laws governing nonprofit institutions. It also allows the state to track its financial healthcare costs better, and; if necessary, regulate the industry. Salary caps can't be instituted on private industries (at this time) by the state. However, to retain a nonprofit status, the state could mandate employees at nonprofits can't make more than $500,000 in total compensation (stocks, bonuses, deferred income, and expenses or benefits), or that the highest salaried employee can't make more than 150% of the least paid employee.

The point would be for states not to end up like the national healthcare programs. For instance, an internal audit of the Pentagon's business operations found $125 billion in annual administrative waste that could be fixed without any job losses or technological upgrades. How much waste is there in paying for-profit companies to administer military healthcare? How much could be re-invested to the nation if these were mandated to be nonprofit subsidies? For perspective, in 2015, Health Net had a gross profit of $2.6 billion, Humana had a gross profit of $10.2 billion, and United Healthcare had a gross profit of $157 billion. How much of that was funded by taxpayer money to Tricare and Medicare? No one knows because those very same companies are fighting the Freedom of Information requests to find out in the courts.

By transitioning to mandatory non-profit industries on the state level, the citizens of that state can see *exactly* where their taxpayer money went to, and how many people directly received care and services, and how much got reinvested into the healthcare system, rather than the pockets of CEOs or shareholders.

Tier Five

While the proposals of Tier Four impact private insurance, they do not directly legislate insurance coverage offered by private insurance or demand corporate change their entire healthcare programs for the state. The following are, in a way, parallel to Tier Four, only targeting Corporate America directly to improve health benefits. In other words, Tier Four and Tier Five could easily be flipped, depending on what proposals states consider a higher priority.

Increased Time Off

Some states, such as California and New York, have already instituted this policy, but more states should follow suit and require mandatory sick time off for all employees. I personally think three days is too little; but it's an excellent start and a great way to promote health while preventing the spread of infection in the workplace. That said, it definitely doesn't go far enough to what states can mandate.

In the universal healthcare systems presented, all have a variant of paid parental leave. It can be up to two years, including splitting the time off between the parents (e.g., one year per parent). Acknowledging two years would never be accepted in the United States either by corporate entities or many individuals, states could mandate corporations provide six months parental leave per parent (for a total of one year) as an excellent start. Corporations will still fight that proposal. However, it is easily economically feasible for companies over 50 employees, whether at full pay or half-pay, if desired.

Another aspect that states could embrace is the understanding of work-life balance. Some nations suggest a four-day work week, which would probably be fine in many states or for many jobs. Another suggestion would be to mandate at least five, preferably fourteen, vacation days. This, like the maternity leave, would be fought tooth and nail by corporate America, but mental health is important to maintain a healthy body, and states requiring vacation time or paid time off can potentially reduce stress-induced illness.

Corporate Coverage
This is actually an adjustment to the current corporate shared cost of medical insurance that exists. Instead of a corporation paying the majority of an insurance plan costs and an employee paying a fraction, a state could mandate that any company with over 50 employees (matching the ACA) is responsible for 100% of the healthcare contract cost with no detriment to employee salary. In other words, instead of a company paying $250 and the employee paying $125 for an insurance policy, the company pays the full amount of $375 and the employee has no deduction on their paycheck.

This would face many court challenges, but legislation should succeed based on the simple fact that these same corporate entities did just this in the 1960s and 70s with little to no reduction to their profits. It helps that many companies not only get huge discounts on bulk insurance plans, but some even get a tax write-off based on additional services offered with the plan: employee wellness, stop smoking initiatives, etc.

This actually provides a stimulus to the economy as employees keep more of their paycheck, puts the onus of healthcare on corporations, and counterbalances the "double dipping" of deals and write-offs companies utilize to pay less in taxes each year. If corporations refuse, thanks to the ACA states can require companies to pay for the ACA Marketplace plans. Of the two options, the Marketplace would probably be more expensive, especially with the patchwork ACA Marketplaces currently instituted across the nation.

Franchise and Corporate Responsibility
This responsibility is based on states requiring corporations and corporate franchises to cover their employees. This is separate from the above proposal, as each individual franchise typically has less than 50 people even if they are contracted with a larger corporate entity. Typically, a franchise like McDonalds or Mail Boxes Etc. has owners offer either insurance coverage by corporate or state healthcare, whichever is cheaper. States could instead require the corporate franchise itself to cover healthcare. There would be legal hoops to jump through, but states have been starting to make corporate owners take more and more responsibility for their franchises.

Another form of *fettering capitalism*, potentially difficult to fight in court, would be for a State to require corporations to pay 100% for employee healthcare insurance unless the average non-manager employee made 30% above the state's minimum wage. In California and Washington, where minimum wage will soon be $15 an hour, this would mean franchises would have to be paying its employees $20 an hour *before* employees are liable for healthcare costs being deducted from their paycheck.

In place of unions fighting for healthcare and better wages, the States force some social engineering on a larger scale, encouraging the multi-billion industries to either pay their employees more or allow said employees to pocket more of their wages while the industries cover healthcare costs. There would be legal challenges, but with the right state and right argument, this could revolutionize both the minimum wage fight and healthcare coverage at once.

Tier Six

Ideally, any or all of the above will have been instituted before states attempt the proposals of this Tier. That said, to build up directly to this Tier, all of **Tier Two** and *Transition to Nonprofits* are the only aspects necessary for these proposals to work, though the rest can only enhance the cost-effectiveness of the proposals. These are effectively state plan outlines, with my own take on how best to maintain self-sustaining systems. This means they do involve cost-sharing, but the tradeoff is a potential state universal healthcare using the systems already in place with just the few tweaks I proposed above.

Medicaid Supplements

This is a partial expansion of Medicaid coverage, and a partial creation of a state-run healthcare plan. It's designed not to impact employers, but expand coverage and decrease costs for patients overall, as well as mitigate the stress of healthcare coverage at trying times of life. It's broken down into three sections.

- The Children's Health Insurance Program (CHIP)
    With the CHIP program integrated into state Medicaid funding, this proposal suggests expanding it from just low-income children, to *all* children from prenatal care through age 18 or when they get their driver's license, whichever is first. This coverage is free for all children. However, if the parents have medical insurance that covers children, the CHIP/Medicaid coverage becomes a *secondary* insurance: it supplements the parents' insurance so the state picks up copays, deductibles, and other costs

that occur with children's healthcare.

The trade-off, however, is that for parents who *do* have commercial insurance and CHIP/Medicaid as a secondary, the parents have an additional 1% to 6% state tax based on single or combined family income. Families who make less than five-times the state or federal poverty level (whichever is higher) would have this tax waived. The tax would help subsidize families who don't have insurance while contributing to the fund's financial health.

- Medicare-Medicaid Plans (Medi-Medi)

Those who are enrolled in the VA, have Medicare, or are Disabled often seek out secondary insurance to help cover the additional costs of Medicare, or for additional coverage (such as dental, vision, etc.). Rather than limit by income those who can benefit from Medicaid as a supplement to Medicare, states should expand affordability and enrollment so Medicare patients can buy-in to Medicaid coverage. This Medicaid plan would cover the Medicare Part A and B deductible, the 20% Medicare Coinsurance, and provide dental, vision, and prescription coverage to some of our most vulnerable members of society. With retirees as the largest growing demographic for the next decade, reducing their financial burden by eliminating the need for expensive supplementary plans will benefit the state economy in the long-run.

For Veterans, the Disabled, and Medicare recipients below 5 times the state poverty level, this could be a free voluntary enrollment. Above that,

Medicare recipients buy-in to the Medicaid coverage on a sliding scale of first dollar amounts (up to $100k income, starting at $25/month, max of $250/month) then percentage based on income (1% at $100k up to 2.5% for over $250k income retirees). As the lower end of the scale some could be paying as little as $100 for coverage that exceeds current supplement plans available, making this a popular potential option.

- Unemployment Insurance

This seems a bit of a no-brainer, but state unemployment should also include healthcare insurance coverage. To that end, those that lose their job and go on unemployment, and don't have expensive COBRA healthcare coverage (continuation of employer insurance through individual payment), should be enrolled in the Medicaid plan. There isn't a buy-in option; the buy-ins from CHIP and Medi-Medi plans would help subsidize this coverage. To ease the stress of keeping this healthcare coverage, this healthcare insurance would last as long as unemployment *plus* one year. If a person is hired by a company, the Medicaid coverage continues for 100 days, as 90 days is the standard employee evaluation and health coverage exemption time in the nation.

Those still unemployed after unemployment and a year, or who don't qualify for unemployment, can enroll on an annual basis, providing proof of non-coverage, non-employment, and inability to afford insurance from other markets (i.e., make less than five times the federal or state poverty level, whichever is highest). This plan would also be open to stay-at-home parents and/or family members not eligible for insurance through other means and for students staying from out-of-state.

Public Option

Unlike the Medicaid option above, which applies only to residents or denizens of a state, a public option can be bought into by employers to cover their associates. Rather than funding from Medicaid, this should instead be financed either through some of the ACA funding states receive to setup marketplaces, or by funding a special project through another state department, such as the Department of Insurance or Department of Agriculture (as is government sponsored farmers insurance), or even funding an independent new state-sponsored nonprofit. However, once the initial setup and network and pharmacy negotiations are complete, this ideally would become a self-funding program as it is not only a buy-in, but has cost sharing as well. Without *fettered capitalism*, cost sharing is the only way to ensure a state healthcare plan doesn't collapse due to excessive costs.

States would have to create provider networks and negotiate on drug prices to create formularies. This could be done as an addendum to the Medicaid negotiations - in which case reimbursement *must* be increased - or the state can attempt to create its own separate negotiations to set up the network. Once these negotiations are complete, states can offer this plan on the statewide exchanges of the ACA, and can even use the pricing for them as a model. Ideally, three plans would be created along the lines of:

- Bronze: 75% coverage, $350 deductible, $7500 Out-of-Pocket max, $55 office copay; cost would be on par with private Bronze plans

- Silver: 85% coverage, $125 deductible, $4800 Out-of-Pocket max, $35 office copay; cost would be between Silver and Gold plans
- Gold: 95% coverage, $0 deductible, $2500 Out-of-Pocket max, $10 office copay; cost would be on par with Platinum plans

These plans would cover at least medical, mental, prescription, vision and dental procedures, though to what extent (i.e., two free dental cleanings, five GP visits, etc.) would have to be determined by the state - with the exception of chronic disease patients, as they will require continual coverage. As pointed out by the federal AmeriCare plan proposal, if a public option like this were available for companies to buy into, within five years the majority would abandon private insurance for the public option. Once again this is a threat to the insurance industry as it stands today, but it could also lead the private insurance industry into competition with the public option, creating better pricing and coverage on the whole for all patients.

Pharmacy Plan
This is similar to the *Public Option* but can be instituted for states who aren't ready to make that final step towards full state-run insurance. Instead, states can set up their own pharmacy benefit plan. This would mean negotiating directly with pharmaceutical companies and offering a public, state plan for pharmacy benefits that citizens and employers could buy into. There would have to be compromises, but this way states can fix drug prices and bypass or co-opt Pharmacy Benefit Managers (PBM) and insurance companies. This gives states the ability to control costs as much as possible.

This sets up the state as a direct competitor, one that PBMs either compete with or lose out. It would mean eliminating the Medicare Part D high costs and non- or partial-coverage that many Medicare patients struggle to afford. It sets a precedent for the state to fix prices for medications that, like Medicare, might set industry price standards in said state. Once a price has been set and accepted, the state could move on to regulating other components' prices, such as medical supplies, hospital treatments, and other healthcare costs - all with a stable public option showing the success of such initiatives.

Dental-Vision Plan

This is identical to the *Pharmacy Plan* above, only instead of the state creating a pharmacy benefit plan, it uses its licensing for vision and dental providers to create a state public option for dental and vision benefits. Perhaps not as high-stakes as drug costs, but when it comes down to vision and dental plans offered nationally, there are far fewer choices and options than healthcare *or* pharmacy benefits. Some offer so little in coverage or reimbursement that despite a monthly cost, patients are effectively uninsured. A state plan would create a new competitor in the market to help set better price standards, and potentially get better coverage across the board. This could be coupled with the *Pharmacy Plan* easily enough as well, and is an excellent stepping stone to either the *Medicaid Supplement* or the full *Public Option*.

Funding Initiatives

Before going in-depth into these proposals, I want to reiterate that these are meant to be paired with any of the above suggestions. However, marrying a funding option to a specific proposal is foolish. A tax that works for one state wouldn't pass in another. So again, please review this as *supplemental* to any of the proposals before, a way to pay for the healthcare initiatives that states could try.

Vice Tax

This is a pretty common tax across states, referring to taxes on products considered a vice, their use not a virtue. For instance, the cigarette tax not only funds anti-smoking measures, but helps dissuade people from smoking. The tax on legal marijuana (for states where it's legal) is another great example of not only taxable income, but *successful* taxable income for a highly sought product that has been a boon to many states.

State alcohol taxes have been stagnant in many states for decades. An additional 1% - 3% tax increase on store-bought and establishment alcohol would bring in millions to billions depending on the state to help fund a healthcare pool. In states where prostitution is legal, a 2% tax increase could have similar results. States that have a lotto could add a 1% annual tax to the accumulated lotto pool earmarked specifically for healthcare. And for gambling states could impose two healthcare taxes: a 0.5% tax on gambling licenses and a 1% tax on the gross profit of gambling locales (casinos, racetracks, etc).

One that might not be thought of as a vice but has been successful in Europe is a sugar tax. Products with a certain percentage of sugar (say above 5%) have an added 3% sales tax - meaning soda and candy could provide a large boost to healthcare funding. As could a 2% tax on all fast food and take-out and/or "Uber" cuisine. Both encourage healthier eating, but as smoking and alcohol taxes have proved, won't result in drastic lower consumption of these products.

Capital Gains & Dividends Tax
Many of the wealthy in the nation get away with paying less in taxes because their income is derived from capital gains and dividends - that is, assets bought and sold and payouts from investments such as stocks and bonds. These are taxed at a lower rate than salary income. Adjusting it to be equal to the standard tax rate of salaried income taxes, even at a state level, could create a revenue of millions to billions, depending on the state. In New York, California, Washington and Texas, this would definitely reach into the billions.

The only question is if this could be taxed at the state level, or if the federal law overrules it. If that's the case, it may be worthwhile for states to institute a tax on all capital gains and dividends. However, if the law was changed nationally, states would lose out, but the nation would gain billions to help offset spending, though maybe not with healthcare.

As an adjunct to this proposal, states could institute a 1 cent fee on all financial transactions and stock purchases; from a single share of stock to a million shares to computer trading. Even a one cent tax on every single high-frequency trade could generate billions per year. Given the billions that these financial institutions make, states could charge a fifty-cent tax per microtransaction with barely an impact on a corporate bottom line.

Employer Contributions

Another item that shouldn't need to be mentioned, the resistance to funding is why it hasn't been suggested: have employers pay directly into a state health fund. Employers already do this on the federal level, with approximately 1% paid by them (and 1% paid by employees) into the federal Medicare fund. A state could implement an additional 1% healthcare tax payable only to the state. Obviously legislation would have to specify that this tax could not affect current salaries - i.e., no lowering employee wages to pay for this - and that 100% liability was on the employers. Using the ACA as a model, those with 50 employees or less would be exempt.

Property Tax Re-Evaluation, a Most Controversial Proposal

In many ways states leave money by the wayside by not re-evaluating locations for taxes. Cities and states, for instance, make deals or bargains with large corporations or sports franchises for corporate, state, and property tax breaks in exchange for an "improved" economy. Some of those deals have paid off, but others - most notably sports arenas and some warehouse stores - have brought a net zero benefit to an area. States could, using this as a basis, revoke those property tax breaks if after a 3- to 5-year period it's shown that the net economic increase promised has not manifested (which is part of why the deals are made).

Corporations would scream, but why provide tax relief to a company that's using valuable property and contributing nothing back to the local economy? If a Walmart fails to provide additional jobs or a boost to the local income, they've obviously not kept up their side of the bargain; even more so if they end up closing the store entirely - the state could demand recompense for the years of uncollected taxes.

Outside of deals, there are many states with archaic rules that have allowed corporate and private industry to pay low property tax despite modern land values. California, for example, has thousands of companies paying property tax from the 1970s, a pittance compared to the millions the land is worth now. The state could institute a re-evaluation of all non-residential property taxes up to a capped percentage and continue to evaluate once every 5 years. In California billions of dollars that could be used for healthcare lay untouched because of corporate and agricultural interests.

And finally, the most controversial would be the re-evaluation of property taxes for nonprofits and religious locales. For nonprofits, the states could review both federal and state regulations and make sure they're adhering strictly to the guidelines. While most would pass muster, plenty of political action committees would be in violation of the social works clause required in some bylaws. Religious institutions would require just as stringent review. Random audits of recorded Sundays to ensure no political proselytizing was going on would have to be conducted, and the removal of televangelists and profit-driven megachurches as "tax exempt" institutions by states would garner some income, but not as much as corporate property tax. When funding healthcare, every penny literally counts towards saving lives.

IN CLOSING

As I stated in the beginning, the single-payer solution isn't impossible, just highly improbable given the circumstances of the system and political realities of our nation. Given time - a generation or three - we could have serious discussions about removing religious objections over scientific fact, accepting we all have skin in the game; and that *fettered capitalism* is essential to affordable healthcare. In fact, some of those discussions are happening right now, but the very powerful and vocal objections are still intruding, are still causing distractions in false statements, and would still rather see people suffer to score political points than for the betterment of the denizens of the United States. Certain States refusing to implement the ACA even after their citizens voted for it via referendum demonstrate that.

While we should look to other nations for inspiration - and, let's be honest, a warning - of how to build and manage healthcare in the future, we are Americans and we should build towards the Holy Grail of single-payer the best way we as a nation have always done: by creating our own melting pot system. It's how we've built our language, our communities, even our governments. Working with wonks, paying attention to nuance, and being aware of the peripheral impacts each decision to transition to new systems is exactly what we need to do to finally, in the future, reach that single-payer grail.

Some work has already been done. The Center for American Progress has come out with a proposal called Medicare <u>Extra</u> For All, which applies universal healthcare, not single-payer, as a stepping stone to get everyone covered, to create a buy-in insurance program with the federal government and regulate drug and procedure pricing. Many of the suggestions I've made above are also part of this proposal.

In addition, a bipartisan commission of Governors has released a Blueprint to Improve the Nation's Health Systems. It's a set of proposed guidelines to follow to try and repair, redirect, and expand the healthcare for the nation. These include expanding what works (i.e., Medicaid expansion), increasing competition among insurers (i.e., break up some of the insurance monopolies), and loosen federal restrictions to encourage creating state-run healthcare systems. Both have aspects I admire and agree with, and both have details I'm concerned about; but they are making the effort, getting the proposals out there and promoting discussions.

There are other initiatives underway that I have reservations about. Amazon, in conjunction with a major investment bank, is looking into entering the healthcare field, either as an insurer, pharmacy, or other facilitator. Though no one can deny the convenience of Amazon, it and its banking partners are primarily focused on profit. As the international review above shows, this is something not usually a part of decent affordable healthcare. Apple is opening its own health kiosks for its employees, where healthcare may be just an app away - but this is also the company that still has labor issues, data privacy scandals, and focuses on lowest cost to produce its products. Uber wants to take over ambulance services, despite its turbulent history and business practices.

On the surface these entities may be disruptive to the healthcare market and may create some lower costs initially; but these are all for-profit corporate entities. They don't tackle the core of the problem nor work towards single-payer. In fact, it fractures the goal of universal healthcare more, rather than trying to improve quality. Nonetheless, given our current healthcare status, we should watch all of these developments very carefully. Perhaps they'll come across some nuance or detail that *does* lead to better and affordable coverage and takes a step towards a better healthcare tomorrow - progress "in spite of" rather than intentionally.

Once again, though, at least these entities are attempting to bring ideas to life, attempting to create a change and bring *discussion* to the forefront of our civil discourse; just as I am attempting to do here. I hope that despite our volatile political situation and the inundation with headlines, memes, and fake news I have brought some understanding to the difficulties in converting suddenly to a single-payer system. I hope I have encouraged and fostered your own thoughts and discussions to occur. Because if we want to save lives and help everyone in the future, we need to begin transforming and improving our healthcare system today.

SOURCES

1. Mossialos, Elias; Djordjevic, Ana; Osborn, Robin; and Sarnak, Dana. "International Profiles of Healthcare Systems." *The Commonwealth Fund.* May 2017.

2. Akhtar, Rais. "Health Care Patterns and Planning in Developing Countries." *Greenwood Press.* 1991. 265 pgs.

3. "Overview of the Spanish Healthcare System." *Imaging Management, Vol. 12, Issue 5.* 2010. Accessed at HealthManagement.org.

4. Puig-junoy, Jaume; Rovira, Joan (June 2004). "Issues raised by the impact of tax reforms and regional devolution on health-care financing in Spain, 1996 - 2002". *Environment and Planning C: Government and Policy.* 22 (3): 453–464.

5. Alfageme, Ana. "Private insurance soars in Spain following cuts to public healthcare." *El Pais.* January 31 2018.

6. U.S. Department of Veterans Affairs (February 9, 2016). "Office of Budget". Va.gov. Retrieved September 20, 2016.

7. U.S. Tricare. "About Us." Tricare.mil. Retrieved August 1, 2018.

8. Monegain, Bernie. "BCBS South Carolina company to process TRICARE claims." *Healthcare IT News.* March 19 2012.

9. Kime, Patricia. "Most beneficiaries satisfied with Tricare, association survey shows." *Military Times.* December 15 2015.

10. Jowers, Karen. "Survey: Troops, families are increasingly dissatisfied with Tricare." *Military Times.* August 2 2018.

11. Cubansky, Juliette and Neuman, Tricia. "The Facts on Medicare Spending and Financing." *Kaiser Family Foundation.* June 22 2018.

12. Rudowitz, Robin and Garfield, Rachel. "10 Things to Know about Medicaid: Setting the Facts Straight." *Kaiser Family Foundation.* April 12 2018.

13. Lipka, Michael and Gramlich, John. "5 Facts About Abortion." *Pew Research Center.* January 26 2017.

14. Bureau of Labor Statistics, State Occupational Employment Statistics Survey, May 2017. *Available at http://www.bls.gov/oes/tables.htm.*

15. Torpey, Elka. "Healthcare: Millions of Jobs Now and in the Future." *Occupational Outlook Quarterly.* Bureau of Labor Statistics. Spring 2014.

16. "US Health Care Spending: A supplement to CHCF's Health Care Costs 101." *California Health Care Foundation.* December 2016.

17. Hamel, Liz; Wu, Bryan; Brodie, Mollyann. "Data Note: Modestly Strong but Malleable Support for Single-Payer Health Care." *Kaiser Family Foundation.* July 5 2017.

18. Chang, Alvin. "Most Bernie Sanders supporters aren't willing to pay for his revolution." *Vox Media.* April 14 2016.

19. Gawande, Atul. "Is Health Care a Right?" *The New Yorker.* October 2 2017. Web.

20. Kliff, Sarah. "What Canada taught Bernie Sanders about health care." *Vox Media.* October